GREEN COFFEE BEAN EXTRACT DIET

Why it Works, How it Works and What You Need to Do For Best Results

There is Hope. There is a Solution...

by J.L. Harper

Green Coffee Bean Extract Diet by J.L. Harper

Copyright 2012

ISBN -13: 978-1479177455

ISBN-10: 1479177458

August 20, 2012, First printing

September 20, 2012Second Printing

September 29, 2012 Third Printing

DEDICATION

To my love, best friend and wife. Thank you for putting up with me for all of these years. Most of all, thank you for finding me!

DISCLAIMER

The claims, information and products mentioned in this book, *Green Coffee Bean Extract Diet,* have not been evaluated by the United States Food and Drug Administration and are not approved to diagnose, treat, cure or prevent disease.

The information provided in the book is for informational purposes only and is not intended as a substitute for advice from your physician or other healthcare professional.

You should not use the information in this book for diagnosis or treatment of any health problem or for prescription of any medication or other treatment.

You should consult with a healthcare professional before starting any diet, exercise or supplementation program, before taking any medication, or if you have, or suspect that you might have a health problem.

The author does not manufacture, sell, distribute green coffee extract, or green coffee.

Introduction

Dr. Oz has put green coffee extract on the front of newspapers, in magazines and has created a buzz in weight loss like we have not seen since the last latest diet fad.

I felt compelled to write this book because it is important for the green coffee extract to not fall in to the abyss with other fad diets due to misuse of the supplement, inferior quality of products and for the few people that will have a difficult time with green coffee extract to ruin it for the vast majority that it will truly work for.

I spoke with a vitamin manufacture the other day and he told me how the price of green coffee extract has tripled since he got his first sample to test. With the popularity of green coffee extract growing at an unprecedented rate it is only a manner of time before inferior and contaminated green coffee extract reaches the market here in America and abroad.

I have turned down a contract with a major book publisher that wanted the rights to my work. They agreed to line up medical experts with all of the proper initials after their name to endorse the book and even have their name on the book as a co-author. A ghost writer was offered if I would just supply the information to write about.

Two things turned me away from a major publisher approach: The book needed to be at least 300 pages in a 6 x 9 size and the book could not give any specific instructions. The book could only give stories of weight loss and not be a manual of what to do and how to do it.

The publisher told me people want stories and really do not care about reading a manual. He went on to tell me "stories sell books" and "manuals gather dust in the bookstore" and "if I wanted to sell books I needed to do it his way or the highway." I have never seen such a look of disgust in my life when I told him I will take the highway.

So, if you want to read stories, there are plenty of stories you can find about green coffee extract on the Internet. You might find some in the reviews section about this book on Amazon or other book selling web sites.

This book is about green coffee bean extract and how you need to take it to be the most effective, why green coffee bean extract works for weight loss, foods you should eat to make the green coffee bean extract be more effective, foods you should avoid if you want the most from green coffee bean extract, and most importantly, to this author anyway, how to use green coffee bean extract and protect your liver.

I hope you enjoy the information in this book, put it to use in your life and lose the weight you have as a goal to lose.

Best,

J.L. Harper

CONTENTS

CHAPTER 1

WHY GREEN COFFEE BEAN EXTRACT WORKS FOR WEIGHT LOSS

The green coffee bean extract has a natural active compound called chlorogenic acid. Too keep this on the simple side, chlorogenic acid is an antioxidant, and it also slows the release of glucose into the blood stream after a meal.

The slowing of glucose release is great but not exactly why green coffee bean extract works for weight loss.

I need to get just a little technical here so try not to go to sleep on me.

We have a gene found in all of our cells that is called the JNK gene. Chlorogenic acid reduces or inhibits this JNK gene from becoming too active. If this JNK gene remains too active for a prolonged period of time weight gain will happen. If you reduce the activity of the JNK gene weight loss will happen.

I so wish I could leave it at that and have this be a "guy" story my family accuses me of telling and preferring but I will give more detail.

You see, I look at the color blue and see blue, I don't see the blue as a shade of other colors blended to make the blue, or look at a portrait and visualize a story and meaning behind what the painter accomplished. This may be boring for some people but it is great for me! I'll do my best to reach the middle ground with this book.

I first ran into this JNK gene while researching for a cause of weight gain being caused by antidepressants. I do quite a bit of research on drugs and this phenomenon of antidepressant induced weight gain could never be nailed down. I want to give you a little more background of how I found this JNK gene and what proceeded afterward.

In 2010, I was taking a break from other research I was conducting and looked to see if anyone had published a study yet that would pinpoint the exact cause of antidepressant induced weight gain. To my pleasant surprise a medical group in Israel just published a study showing the cause of antidepressant weight gain. (1) In this study they mentioned the JNK gene as the starting point for obesity as well as weight gain caused by antidepressants.

I then did an Internet search regarding the JNK gene and came across a study conducted by Harvard School of Public Health, November 2002, which detailed how the JNK gene directly affected weight gain and how it could be used for weight loss. The Harvard School of Public Health has titled their study, *Key Gene Discovered for Obesity and Diabetes*. (2)

After reading the Harvard study I felt it was only a matter of time before a drug company produced a weight loss drug and proceeded to search to see if one was under way. I ran into patents issued to a drug discovery company Celgene and reading through their patent I noticed it covered not only reducing the activation of the JNK gene but for the treatment of diabetes, obesity, Parkinson's, cancer and a host of other diseases, illnesses and conditions.

After seeing all of this information I searched a list of all clinical studies and found these diseases, illnesses and conditions had as a root the over activation of this JNK gene. Many of the studies show if the JNK gene activation is reduced the disease, illness and condition went away. How interesting is that? Hopefully, this has your attention a little more now and it might make more sense why I would not just write a book about weight loss and only have stories inside.

I then began to research and found several studies showing natural substances, foods, supplements and more that would reduce the over activation of the JNK gene. This led down several interesting twists and turns and brought up the origin of the JNK where it was first thought to only be an enzyme. The real application of the JNK information requires the information be used to increase or decrease the JNK enzymes as well as to increase or decrease the activation of the gene.

The enzyme JNK3 affects the brain, heart and testis, the JNK2 affects the skin and the JNK1 affects all other parts of the body. Science has narrowed this down to the point where it is known the JNK3 enzyme becomes over activated when an opiate or pain killer is taken. The

JNK3 enzyme kills brain cells and this is the starting point of the side effects associated with pain killers and what leads to further degeneration of the brain.

Long story short: I have had amazing results with naturally reducing the over activation of the JNK gene and JNK enzymes and that is what the green coffee bean extract is doing and why it is effective for weight loss.

Don't be surprised along the way if you experience complete body resurgence and your mental functioning blossoms as well. Natural supplements are being used with success for the treatment of dementia, clinical studies conducted at U. Mass. Lowell, have shown remarkable success and the underlying natural treatment has been addressing the JNK.

My initial theory was; the green coffee bean extract is inhibiting the JNK1 pathway and will probably not be helping the brain at all by directly inhibiting the JNK3. However, with the green coffee bean extract also regulating glucose and inflammation you will have a byproduct that ultimately helps how you feel mentally when these are relieved.

My theory of the JNK1 has now been confirmed and published in Journal of Agricultural and Food Chemistry, paid for by Kraft Foods Research. Green coffee been extract does inhibit the JNK1 and the JNK2. With the JNK2 being confirmed, don't be surprised if you see a skin cream with green coffee bean extract as the main ingredient in the future. If you inhibit JNK2, skin cancer will not start or continue to exist.

CHAPTER 2

THE TYPE OF GREEN COFFEE BEAN EXTRACT TO USE

Green coffee bean extract is a coffee bean, at least when you plant the seed.

Selecting the right green coffee bean extract supplement should be judged on:

- Milligrams per capsule (400 mg is ideal)
- Make sure it has 50% chlorogenic acid
- Make sure the product is independently tested for strength
- Make sure the product is independently tested for purity
- Make sure it is decaffeinated
- Price should be last

It is easy to look at the label and read if the capsules are 400 mg and if the chlorogenic acid content is at 50%. The company selling it should be proud of the chlorogenic acid content and advertise it on the label.

The next qualifications can be a little trickier to verify. The highest standard for a vitamin manufacture is to be what is called cGMP certified. This is where the F.D.A. comes in to the facility and inspects the manufacturing plant; the testing procedures used and give their ongoing stamp of approval.

Most supplements sold are done as a private label and the company making the supplement is not the company that sells to the end user. This is where you can find quality dropping off sharply. Bottles of green coffee bean extract might be manufactured in China and residue of Prozac or other drugs can be found in the capsules.

The best solution to avoid this is to purchase from the manufacture that states they are Made in America and cGMP certified.

CHAPTER 3

HOW TO TAKE GREEN COFFEE BEAN EXTRACT FOR WEIGHT LOSS

First Week

Take 800 mg's first thing in the morning.

Take an additional 800 mg's every 4 hours throughout the day and evening. **This may require 2 capsules of the 400 mg capsule.**

You need to keep the JNK gene from becoming over activated during the day and night for the maximum weight loss.

Studies have not shown how long the green coffee bean extract will keep the JNK gene in check but by other studies with other supplements and drugs, my best guess is 4 hours.

You can certainly try the recommend dosages used by Dr. Oz but if you are taking the right green coffee bean extract and weight loss does not start within the second week, it is time to use the dosages and the amount I am suggesting.

Reversing insulin resistance needs to be accomplished. If you are taking or ever used an antidepressant, you are insulin resistant, no question. One week of the **First Week** approach should handle this and then you are ready to start losing weight.

Second Week

Now you can reduce the green coffee extract down to 400 mg per serving but keep taking a capsule every 4 hours throughout the day.

Third Week

As long as you are now losing at least 2 pounds each week, reduce the green coffee bean extract to 1 capsule 30-minutes before each meal. Take at least 3 capsules a day whether a meal is eaten or not.

Take 1 capsule in the morning, 1 more around noon and 1 more any time after 6 pm.

CHAPTER 4

FOODS YOU SHOULD EAT MORE OF

I understand the hype on the green coffee bean extract; you can eat whatever you want and not exercise and still lose weight. This will be true for some people but not for all dieters. The reviews on Amazon.com already show this.

If you want to get the most out of taking the green coffee you will do as much as possible to keep the JNK gene reduced.

Eat plenty of vegetables, the darker the better to help stop the over activation of the JNK gene. Fruit, especially the skin, darker the better, inhibits the JNK gene. You do not need to be a vegetarian, but eat more fruit and veggies!

If you are starting to think this is like any other diet, slow down the mind and keep reading. Of course if you eat a gallon of ice cream at bedtime and junk food all day and are 200 pounds overweight, eating nothing but veggies and fruit all day will cause weight loss and probably make you jump off a bridge in the process.

Try eating more fresh veggies and try snacking on fruit as well. This is a healthy suggestion as well as one for weight loss.

You do not starve yourself. If you do, the JNK gene will remain over activated and beyond the loss of muscle mass you will not lose weight or size. I have had to help too many people that used the Hcg diet regain their health. Eating 500 calories a day puts the body in starvation mode and the drug itself plays havoc on all systems of the body.

Eat   to   Survive   -   Do   not   Survive   to   Eat

Not all of us have a problem with portion size, so I will not harp on that further. Just know, if you leave the dinner table and you are stuffed, you have eaten too much for sure, and probably the wrong foods if they were not fruits, veggies and a small portion of meat.

These foods and spices will help inhibit the JNK gene:

- Almonds
- Cayenne pepper
- Cloves

- Curcumin

- Garlic (Fresh garlic only. Thirty minutes or less before meal preparation, press fresh garlic. Using garlic in any other manner or a non-fresh garlic will have the reverse effect)

- Ginger (Use as spice or drink at least 2 cups of ginger tea each day)

- Green Tea Extract (a cup or 2 of green tea each day)

- Omega 3 fish oil (at least 2,000 mg of pure fish oil daily. Omega 3 fish oil will deplete vitamin E from the body. Supplementing with 200 i,u, of vitamin E daily is recommended if taking fish oil)

- Oranges

- Papaya

- Paprika

- Red Pepper

- Reishi

- Tomato (the skin is the important part of the tomato for JNK reduction)

- Vegetables

- Eat lean meats, plenty of vegetables and fruit.

These are the foods most healthcare providers claim we should have more of. Reducing the activation of the JNK gene is why these foods are great for our body. This may not seem like new information to most of you but it is new information regarding what these foods are actually doing.

If your diet is terrible, bring them in gradually or you may have too much of a shock to your system.

Eating meat that is free of antibiotics and hormones will also help keep the JNK gene from being over activated.

Try eating these foods for 2 or 3 days straight, if you are new to this type of food. Then eat as you were doing and then come back again. It gets a lot easier with time.

CHAPTER 5

FOODS YOU SHOULD AVOID

As much as possible, cut out:

- **Preservatives** in the food

- Limit dairy. You just need to limit the amount of dairy from what you currently consume.

- Refined sugar

- White bread

- **Frozen fish** (Fresh fish that you freeze at home is fine but NO frozen fish from a store. The preservatives that are used are the worst of the worst)

Datum's to use:

- If the food makes you feel **very** full, it is the wrong food for you.

- If the food makes you get bloated, it is the wrong food for you

- If you finish a meal and you are still hungry, you either need to eat more or it is the wrong food for you. You do not want to starve the body. Weight loss will stop if you do.

- You should feel the need for additional nourishment around 2 hours after your last meal. This is the time to have a light snack. Try raw veggies, almonds, some fruit or yogurt.

For most American's canned goods are a way of life but in fact, they are a way toward death. If you stand in a grocery store and watch what people are buying, the canned goods section is packed.

It can take 10-days to change a habit and the same holds true with food selection. Make your food list before going to the store and stick with it completely.

Organic milk cost more to buy but if you reduce the amount of milk you consume the cost averages out. The hormones and antibiotics found in other milk will activate the JNK gene and make weight loss more difficult.

The same holds true for meat. Meat filled with preservatives, hormones and antibiotics activate the JNK gene.

The same holds true for eggs.

CHAPTER 6

FREE FATTY ACIDS

Most diets fail and people give up due to free fatty acids.

When you lose weight the fatty acids begin to leave your cells. This is a good thing and is part of size reduction and the weight loss. With the fatty acids now out of the cells and in the bloodstream they are now called free fatty acids. The fatty acids are called free because they are no longer attached to anything.

The body begins to have a difficult time moving the free fatty acids out and the free fatty acids begin to build up in the liver. The free fatty acids activate the JNK gene and weight loss stops. When a person is 50-pounds overweight and they restrict calories and what they eat for 7 days, weight loss will happen during the first week but right around the first part of week two the weight loss stops. This should not be the case with a person that much overweight. The reason is due to the fatty acids and the JNK gene becoming over activated again.

On top of the JNK gene becoming over activated again and weight loss stopping, the person will begin to develop **non-alcoholic fatty liver disease**. It is estimated one third of the population of the United States has **non-alcoholic fatty liver disease.** This should not be a surprise with around twenty five percent of the population being obese or overweight, dieting by that population in an attempt to lose the weight and free fatty acids creating **non-alcoholic fatty liver disease** and the activation of the JNK in the liver.

Having problems with your gull bladder? The JNK enzyme called JNK1 increases liver cell death by the toxic bile acid called deoxycholate. The obesity rate of kids and teens has been on the rise for enough time now and gull bladder removal for this age group has followed the upward trend.

You are probably getting the idea now of what has been happening inside your body every time you have been on a diet. You do some things that are excellent for your health with a food change or calorie restriction but the unseen damage takes place in the liver, gull bladder and other parts of the body; weight loss stops and on top of that the liver has now taken the hit.

You might be asking yourself at this point, why don't doctors know of the JNK gene, free fatty acids and other things I am writing about in this book? If your doctor graduated from medical school before 2002, they never would have heard about the JNK gene. Talking with several physicians that just completed their schooling, most remembered hearing something about a gene called JNK but they did not recall the specifics.

Specialists in their given field do know about the JNK gene and the link between obesity and most other diseases. Until they have a drug to sell or find some way to make money with the information, the JNK gene information will not be known broadly. The first JNK drug will probably be approved by the F.D.A. around 2016, and it will be heralded as the new wonder drug. Nature has given us the way to handle the JNK with natural means.

Source: Harper's Biochemistry, 25th Edition, Appleton & Lance, Stanford, Connecticut, 2000, Page 302

"The liver plays a regulatory role in removing excess free fatty acids from the circulation."

"However in the face of an increased influx of free fatty acids, an alternative route, ketogenosis, is available that enables the liver to continue to retransport much of the influx of free fatty acids in a form readily utilized by extrahepatic (non-liver tissues) tissues under all nutritional conditions."

"as more fatty acid is oxidized, more forms ketone bodies and less forms CO_2."

I will end here before I get into write a book on biochemistry. The point is, the green coffee bean extract can do a remarkable job of allowing fatty acids to flow from the cells and become free at last. However, and I need to get a little philosophical with this, when you free something it must be freed into something else. How many times over the past few thousand years have we read about freedom of a country or a group. The excitement that follows is tremendous. However, if some other structure is not instantly put in place the people begin to turn on each other and destroy the country or the group. Look at the middle-east right now with dictators being thrown out or killed. The population is now free of the dictator but in the case of Libya the people are beginning to turn on each other.

Egypt is a great example to use for free fatty acids. The people wanted a change from their dictator and they got that. Now their freedom from that is like a free fatty acid and the start of **non-alcoholic fatty liver disease.**

The body tends to mimic society. Cells will steal from other cells, cells will kill off weak cells and steal their bounty, cells will remember what was done to them and concoct a plan to get even and the list goes on and on. Sometimes I wonder if the cells are mimicking us or are we mimicking our cells. At least we would be making a cognitive decision to do something, whether we are aware of the decision or not. Otherwise the placebo effect would not exist.

This is definitely moving away from free fatty acids in this chapter but I am rolling and don't want to stop. This past year the F.D.A. has approved a new diet drug. Looking through the clinical studies on the drug, one interesting thing pops out, placebo effect. You might think a drug for weight loss would be like setting a fractured bone. It is either set or not set and is proved by an x-ray. If a weight loss drug has a placebo effect and people can lose nearly as much weight with a placebo as they do with the drug, our own mind has some control over weight loss.

We might live in a world where shades of gray are everywhere but there is no shade of gray here. If the mind did not control weight loss to some degree we would not have seen any placebo effect during the weight loss drug studies. Some will want to argue with me on this point the same way it was argued the earth must be flat because it looks flat.

Start picturing you as thinner and it just might help. Lose 5 pounds and admire the body for the accomplishment and it just might help. I doubt seriously if a person that is 50 pounds overweight can simply will their way to losing the 50-pounds by some magical thought. However, can they help the process out in some manner, yes they can or there would not be a placebo effect with weight loss drugs.

Stress activates the JNK gene. Getting all stressed by how you look, stressed by not fitting in your clothes only compounds the situation.

CHAPTER 7

HOW TO FLUSH FREE FATTY ACIDS

There is several ways to assist the liver in removing free fatty acids.

Acetyl-L-carnitine - Acetyl-L-carnitine is an amino acid and helps the body produce energy. This amino acid also helps reduce the over activation of the JNK gene. The United States Army conducted a clinical study with acetyl-L-carnitine to see if it might help with hearing loss due to loud noises. The studies were promising as they should be if a supplement reduced the activation of the JNK. Take 1,000 mg in the morning and 1,000 mg mid-afternoon.

CoQ10 - CoQ10 helps burn fat while it is still inside the cells. Not a bad thing. Taking 100 mg a day would be the right amount.

Milk Thistle - Milk thistle is known as a natural liver healer and will also help remove fatty acid buildup. Around 250 mg in the morning and 250 mg in the evening works the best.

JNK Liquid Booster – (*The JNK Liquid Booster is sold at Amazon.com. Just type in the Amazon search box, JNK Liquid Booster. The manufacture is TRB Health. I do not distribute, sell or manufacture the JNK Liquid Booster*) One supplement mixture I have recommended for years is called JNK Liquid Booster. The independent clinical studies with the JNK Liquid Booster show what should be happening when free fatty acids are addressed in the liver as well as a further reduction of liver JNK. The clinical studies are below:

(1) The **first study** shows:

This first study was made to see if the nutrient concentrate could improve lipid (fat) metabolism at a very early stage of being overweight. This study also had no dietary modifications other than using the nutrient concentrate in lieu of breakfast.

My observation: The weight loss is ok but the reduction of blood pressure, cholesterol LDL, triglycerides, blood glucose reduction, insulin reduction, SGOT and SGPT activity decrease is better than you will find with any medication.

Weight loss: 4% (5.72 lbs)
Waist size reduction: 5.4% (1.73in)
Buttocks size reduction: 2.6% (0.94 in)
Rump size reduction: 3.2% (1.18in)
Blood pressure reduction: 1.6%
Total cholesterol reduction: 4.7%
LDL cholesterol reduction: 2.0 %
Triglycerides reduction: 29.5%
Blood glucose reduction: 12.1%

Insulin reduction: 12.6%

SGOT activity decrease: 1.4 %

SGPT activity decrease: 3.3%

Influence of a liquid nutrient concentrate on lipid metabolism parameters in slightly overweight individuals.

Anatoly. G. Antoshechkin, M.D., Ph.D

Scientific Director, Genext Research, Inc.

Abstract

A nutrient concentrate was studied for its ability to influence on some clinical manifestations that are characteristic of changes in lipid metabolism. Such studies usually focus on individuals who are significantly overweight or obese. In this study, however, participants were selected to form a group of individuals who were only slightly overweight, as indicated by an average body mass index (BMI) of 25.2.

35 healthy adults (26 females and 9 males) ingested the nutrient concentrate instead of breakfast for 36 days. They were instructed to make no other changes to their life styles. The participants made no modifications to their lunches or dinners but ate the food they normally would eat.

Measurements of blood pressure, concentration of glucose, insulin, two liver enzymes, total cholesterol, LDL, HDL, triglycerides and certain anthropometric measurements were carried out before and after the trial.

The most significant results of the trial are reduction of blood triglyceride levels– 29.5% of the initial concentration. In individuals with increased blood insulin level (hyperinsulinemia), the average decrease of initial level was 22.0%. Blood sugar, insulin and cholesterol levels also decreased.

An unexpected result was a reduction in the activity of two liver enzymes (SGOT and SGPT). This indicates that the nutrient concentrate may have a systemic cleansing or detoxifying effect.

Body weight and body size measurements were also significantly reduced.

Introduction

Few people, who are concerned about and pay attention to their body weight, realize that being overweight is manifestation of a disturbed lipid metabolism. In order to be able to control ones weight, it is necessary to influence the state of one's lipid metabolism.

The beginning of weight gain is usually accompanied by changes of lipid metabolism. An important manifestation of weight gain in an increase in the circumference of the waist.

Harvard Medical School doctors recommend:

"Rather than being an endorsement for getting fat, these findings may help us to pay attention to our waists, in addition to our weight. For most of us, the plain fact is that weight gain when we're adults is an indication that we are, indeed, getting fatter and therefore very likely at greater risk of suffering from a long list of diseases.

It does get a little more complicated in older age. We lose muscle mass and bone density, so while we may weigh the same as we used to, or even less (and congratulate ourselves on being thin), we may actually be lugging around more fat tissue. So we need to keep an eye on our waist size, not just our weight, especially after about age 50. Waist size is a fairly accurate reflection of how much visceral fat we've accumulated in our abdomens. And visceral fat is the metabolically active form of fat that causes so much harm" (1).

In most studies dedicated to weight loss by dieting, participants are either significantly overweight or obese. Our study examines the beginning stage of weight gain and on the changes in lipid metabolism indicators that are reflected by blood analysis.

The trial participants, dietary conditions and examinations

35 adult healthy individuals (26 females and 9 males) participated in the trial. They were only marginally overweight, with an average Body Mass Index of 25.2 (normal range is 18.5 - 24.9). In fact, the BMI of the participants bordered on normal.

During the trial, which lasted 36 days, the participants took a liquid nutrient concentrate instead of eating breakfast. They were instructed to make no other changes to their life styles. The participants made no modifications to their lunches or dinners but ate the food they normally would eat. Following the trial, the participants were questioned regarding any side effects experienced during the trial.

In each participant, the following measures were carried out before and after the trial: blood pressure, two liver enzymes SGOT and SGPT, determination in the blood the levels of following indicators of lipid metabolism: glucose, insulin, total cholesterol, low density lipoproteins (LDL), high density lipoproteins (HDL), triglycerides and some anthropometric measurements.

Results

Measurements carried out before and after the trial showed the following average changes for the 35 participants:

WEIGHT REDUCTION

WEIGHT LOSS: 2.6 kg (4.0% reduction)

SIZE REDUCTIONS

NECK: 0.67 cm (1.9 % reduction)

CHEST: 1.89 cm (2.1% reduction)

WAIST: 4.4 cm (5.4% reduction)

BUTTOCKS: 2.4 cm (2.6% reduction)

RUMP: 2.99 cm (3.2% reduction)

BLOOD ANALYSIS

BLOOD PRESSURE REDUCTION: 2.06/1.09 (1.6% reduction)

TOTAL CHOLESTEROL REDUCTION: 9.51 mg/dL (4.7% reduction)

LDL REDUCTION: 4.15 mg/dL (2.0 % reduction)

HDL REDUCTION: 0.13 mg/dL (0.2% reduction)

TRIGLYCERIDES REDUCTION: 35.14 mg/dL (29.5% reduction)

BLOOD GLUCOSE REDUCTION: 11.5 mg/dL (12.1% reduction)

INSULIN REDUCTION: 1.06 IU/ml (12.6% reduction)

SGOT ACTIVITY DECREASE: 0.34 U/L (1.4 % decrease)

SGPT ACTIVITY DECREASE: 0.91 U/L (3.3% decrease)

The results obtained show that the intake of the nutrient concentrate during 36 days instead of a normal breakfast reduces the indicated parameters. The most significant changes concern weight, waist size and triglycerides.

It should be noted that the influence of the nutrient concentrate appears more effective in an individual with elevated blood concentration of triglycerides, total cholesterol, insulin and LDL before the trial since these readings in such individuals showed a greater reduction following the trial.

In five individuals with high level of triglycerides in blood (more 200 mg/dL, ranging from 230 to 315 mg/dL), the average reduction of the concentration of triglycerides was 163.4 mg/dL—60% of the average level of triglycerides before the trial in these five participants.

In 17 individuals with level of total cholesterol in the blood higher than 200 mg/dL,(ranging from 200 to 304 mg/dL), the average reduction of the initial level was 21.8 mg/dL —10% of the average level in these 17 persons before the trial.

In three participants with high blood levels of LDL (more 160 mg/dL, ranging from 126 to 176 mg/dL), the average LDL reduction was 36 mg/dL—23% of the initial concentration of LDL before the trial.

In eight persons with increased blood insulin level (higher than 10 IU/ml, ranging from 10.5 to 20.3 UI/ml), the average decrease of the initial level was 3.2 IU/ml—a 22.0% of the initial level in these eight participants before the trial. In others participants concentration of insulin in the blood before the trial was on normal level and changed insignificantly.

An unexpected result was a reduction in the liver enzyme activity (1.4% reduction in SGOT and 3.3% reduction in SGPT), which indicates that the nutrient concentrate may have a systemic cleansing or detoxifying effect.

As evidenced by the questionnaire that the participants filled out following the program, no comments were made by the participants during the trial indicating side effects such as feeling week or hungry.

Discussion

The participants in this trial do not belong to a typical overweight category. Their BMI was an average of 25.2, which is bordering on normal. Nevertheless, the intake of the nutrient concentrate during the trial demonstrates a significant influence on lipid metabolism and body weight.

It is important to note that the nutrient concentrate was used only once per day instead of eating a usual breakfast. The participants made no other modifications to the food intake during the rest of the day (lunch and dinner), nor did they in any other way change their life styles.

It is not surprising that in patients with higher levels of triglycerides, total cholesterol, LDL and insulin the decrease of these blood components was more significant. The greater the lipid metabolism misbalance, the more remarkable can be the influence of an effective remedy to normalize metabolic balance.

The effect of the nutrient concentrate could be explained by the following factors:

(1) A substitution of breakfast with a liquid nutrient concentrate reduces the intake of calories and cholesterol.

(2) Constituents in the nutrient concentrate may reduce appetite and therefore also decrease the intake of substances such as cholesterol.

(3) Some plant compounds in the nutrient concentrate may modulate expression of genes involved in lipid metabolism. The ability of some herbal extracts to influence on gene expression has been demonstrated in experiments with cultivated human cells (2, 3).

There is also recent evidence of gene-nutrient interactions with dietary fat (4).

The results obtained in this trial point to a recommendation to control lipid metabolism during the beginning stage of the development of gaining weight. Even with a BMI near 25, the use of a remedy that is capable of normalizing deviations from norm in lipid metabolism, such as the nutrient concentrate used in this study, should be recommended.

References

(1) HealthBeat, Harvard Medical School, Issue May 25, 2010.

(2) Antoshechkin A, Olalde J, Magarici M. et al. **Analysis of effects of the herbal preparation Circulat on gene expression levels in cultured human fibroblasts.** *Phytother Res. 2007; 21: 777-89.*

(3) Antoshechkin A, Olalde J, Antoshechkina M et al. **Influence of the plant extract complex "AdMax" on global gene expression levels in cultured human fibroblasts.**

J Diet Suppl. 2008; 5: 293-304.

(4) Phillips CM, Goumidi L, Bertais S et all. **Gene-nutrient interactions with dietary fat modulate the association between genetic variation of the ACSL1 gene and metabolic syndrome.** *J Lipid Res. 2010 Feb 22 [Epub].*

(2) This **second study** results show:

Weight loss: 7.5 lbs
Body fat percentage reduction: 3.02%
Waist size reduction: 2.32 inches
Hips size reduction: 2.80 inches
Chest size reduction: 1.93 inches
Abdomen size reduction: 2.45 inches
Glucose reduction: 3.17 mg/dL
Total cholesterol reduction:5 mg/dL
Triglycerides reduction: 22.31 mg/dL

Effect of a short term nutrient concentrate program on weight management, adipose tissue, cholesterol and triglycerides in overweight adults.

Michael J. Gonzalez, Jorge R. Miranda-Massari, Carlos M. Ricart, Heidi Ortega and Saisha M. Muñiz Alers

InBio Med Projec, Medical Sciences Campus School of Public Health and Pharmacy and Dept. of Biology Cayey Campus, University of Puerto Rico.

Abstract

A nutrient concentrate consisting of a liquid supplement and a protein supplement was studied to determine its safety and efficacy on weight/fat loss, cholesterol and triglycerides levels in thirty five overweight adults between ages 14-60.

This open label trail measured total body weight, body fat percentage, waist circumference, hips (females), chest (females), abdomen (males), glucose, total cholesterol and triglycerides before and after one week on the concentrate.

A group of thirteen subjects continued on the concentrate for one more week and anthropometric measures were obtained. Interestingly after only one week on the program the subjects experience a statistically significant ($p < 0.05$) weight reducing effect. This weight reduction was accompanied with a corresponding statistically significant ($p < 0.05$) decrease in body fat percentage.

In addition a significant decrease in total cholesterol ($p < 0.05$) and triglycerides ($p < 0.01$) resulted.

Also reduction in waist, hip and chest measurements were obtained. We conclude that the nutrient concentrate and protein supplement program studied herein is a safe and effective way to assist adults in weight, fat, cholesterol and triglyceride reduction.

Introduction

The public health problem of obesity and unhealthy weight gain has grown considerably in the United States in recent years (1). We know this is a chronic disease that involves complex interactions among genetics, environmental, cultural and behavioral factors. A positive energy balance is required in order for weight gain to occur. In other words energy intake must exceed energy expenditure.

Obesity is among the easiest medical conditions to diagnose, but most difficult to treat. The annual cost to society for obesity is estimated to be at nearly $ 100 billion/year (2). Moreover, unhealthy weight gain is responsible for over 300,000 deaths/ year (3). Obesity has serious health consequences that have a disproportionate effect on minorities, women, children, the aged population and those in lower socioeconomic status. Obesity is associated with type II Diabetes mellitus, it increases the risk for Coronary Heart Disease, Osteoarthritis, Cancer and Stroke (4). We embarked in this study to evaluate the safety and efficacy of this short term dietary supplement program for weight/ fat loss.

Methods

The target subjects included overweight and obese (10% and above average body weight with a body mass index (BMI) over 25. The study sample consisted of 35 experimental subjects for the first week and 13 follow up experimental subjects for the second week those consisted of 22 females and 13 males between the ages of 14-60 in the first group and 13 subjects that decided to continue the diet for one more week (10 females and 3 males) in the second group.

All participants completed a general health questionnaire and anthropological measures such as body weight, height, percent body fat, waist, hip, and chest measurements. Blood tests (fasting) such as CBC and SMA 20 were taken at the beginning of the study and a week after treatment. Eligible volunteers meeting all inclusion criteria who consented were included in the study and provided with the supplements. The participants received a liquid nutrient concentrate to be utilized for a week as part of the experimental program.

This product consisted of a blend of juices including aloe and pomegranate and mixture of botanical tea extracts that included Ginseng, Green tea, Gymmena silvestre, Garcinia cambodia, Yerba mate, Cascara sagrada, plus a mixture of additional vitamins and minerals, (B complex, Vitamin C and Chromium).

For the purpose of controlling the calorie intake during the study and ensure that the participants a balanced diet, they also received a protein shake consisting of 16g of protein, 1g of fat, 1g of sugar, 2g of fiber and an enzyme mixture per serving. The participants were recommended to take the protein shake twice a day with skim milk as breakfast and lunch. The participants were encouraged to do some form of daily exercise, such as a half hour walk. They were otherwise instructed to continue their normal lifestyle with no other weight reduction regime other than the experimental program. Compliance with all study related procedures were strictly monitored. All subjects dispensed with enough concentrate and protein for a week of use.

Statistical analysis

The data was analyzed using the statistical package SPSS version 12. A Kolmogorov-Smirnoff goodness of fit test was performed on all variables in the experimental group to test the null hypothesis that the data came from a normally distributed population. The results accepted the null hypothesis for all variables ($p < 0.05$). Next a parametric paired-sample t-test was carried out to determine that there is no significant difference between the mean of the initial measurements (i.e. before treatment) and the mean of the subsequent measurements (i.e post-treatment).

This test was performed for each variable included in the exper mental group (treated with the dietary program). All results rejected the null hypothesis and the means were significantly different (p< 0.05). Also an analysis of variance was performed between the three measurements resulting in a significant difference (p < 0.05) among the three measurements. Finally, a Pearson coefficient was calculated to test the degree of correlation in the change detected between the pre and post-treatments. All results showed a significant coefficient (p<0.05) consistent with the changes observed experimentally.

Results

All measurements reported on the 36 subjects were taken twice during the study (at the beginning and at 7 days of dietary treatment) another measurements were taken on the 13 subjects that continued treatment for one more week. All subjects served as their own controls.

Total body weight: The average weight loss was 7.5 lb. ± 2.30 during one week of dietary treatment. The mean ± SE per body weight at the beginning of the study was 198.34 lb. ± 6.68 and at the end of the week was 190.89 lb. ± 6.21. This difference was found to be statistically significant (p < 0.05). In the 13 subjects that continued the dietary program for 1 more week their mean body weight after the treatment was 180.52 lb. ± 5.51 (their mean body weight before second treatment was 188.55 lb. ± 4.87)

Body Fat Percentage: The average % fat loss was 3.02% ± 0.99. The mean ± SE for body fat % at the beginning of the study was 39.61% ±

1.07 and at the end was 36.59% ± 1.01. This difference was found to be significant (p < 0.05). In the subjects that extended their treatment for one more week the mean body fat percentage was 33.01% ± 0.98 (The man body fat percentage before the second treatment was 36.20% ± 1.01).

Waist measurement: The average waist measurement loss was 2.32 in ± 0.81. The waist measurement at the beginning was 40.046 in ± 1.03 and at the end 38.14 in ±0.99. This difference was found to be significant (p < 0.05). The subjects that followed treatment for one more week the mean waist measurement was 36.25 in ± 1.01 (Their mean measurement before the second treatment was 38.29 in ± 1.01).

Hips measurement: This measurement was only taken on females. The average hip measurement loss was 2.80 in ± 1.05. The mean hip measurement at the beginning was 44.89 in ± 1.07 and at the end of the first week 42.09 in ± 1.00. In the subjects that had an extra week of the treatment the mean was 40.20 in ± 0.99. These differences were found to be statistically significant (p<0.05).

Chest measurement: This measurement was also taken just on female subjects. The average chest measurement at the beginning of the study was 42.04 in ± 1.08 and at the end 40.11 in ± 1.07. In the subjects that furthered their treatment for a week the mean was 37.98 in ± 1.05.These differences were statistically significant (p<0.05).

Abdomen measurement: The measurement was done only on male subjects. The average loss on abdomen measurement was 2.45 in ± 0.99. The abdomen measurement at the beginning of the study was 44.00 in ± 1.02 and at the end 41.66 in ± 0.88. For the group that had an extra week of treatment the average measurement was 38.42 in ± 0.90. These differences were found to be statistically significant.

Glucose: Glucose measurement at the beginning of the study was 84.99 mg/dL ± 1.47 and at the end 81.82 mg/dL ± 1.43. For the group that had an extra week of treatment was 80.75 ± 1.45.

Here a tendency toward reduction was attained but only statistical difference was obtained for the pretreatment vs. post treatment values ($p < 0.05$).

Total cholesterol: The average loss of total cholesterol was 5 mg/dL ± 5.25. The total cholesterol at the beginning was 186.32mg/dL ± 7.85 and at the end 181.32 mg/dL ± 0.81. For the group that had an extra week of treatment was 180.37 mg/dL ± 4.55. These differences did not result in a statistical difference. Nevertheless, when we separate the subjects that had total cholesterol over 200 from the rest of the group (14 subjects) their total cholesterol at the beginning was 237.5 mg/ dL ± 5.51 and at the end it was 211.05 mg/dL ± 5.25 which resulted in a statistically significant difference ($p < 0.01$).

Triglycerides: The average loss in triglyceride value was 22.31 mg/dL ± 7.01. The triglyceride level at the beginning of the study was 115.25 mg/dL ± 9.52 and the end was 92.94 mg/dL ± 7.09. The triglyceride level for the subject that had an extra week of treatment was 80.37 mg/dL ±6.99. These differences had a statistical significance ($p < 0.05$).

Discussion

This clinical investigation utilizing a short term nutrient concentrate and protein supplement program for weight/fat loss was undertaken because to date data available on safety and efficacy of such programs are lacking. Most short term "fad" diets may produce weight loss by means of solely water loss with no measurable fat loss.

This research was an open label experimental clinical trial in which subjects served as their own control for a period of one week and a subset for another additional week. The primary aim of the research was to test for the program safety and the secondary aim was to test for effectiveness by identifying any changes in total body weight, body fat percentage, waist, hips, chest measurements, as well as glucose, total cholesterol and triglycerides. In relation to total body weight, we achieved a significant reduction in only seven days on the program.

Moreover, body fat percentage was significantly reduced during that short period. These results demonstrated in part that weight loss was due to fat loss instead of only water content or muscle loss. Waist, hips, abdomen, and chest measurements were also significantly reduced.

These results are of great importance to the subjects since the loss of fat inches is what they perceive as success rather than just the loss of body weight. Also 90% of the subjects reported reduce appetite and more energy while in the program. There was a tendency of reduction of fasting blood glucose but did not reach statistical significance although we should mention that fasting blood glucose in the subjects at the start of the study were within normal ranges. The only statistical difference was obtained when comparing pre-treatment vs. post-treatment. We should state this difference was within normal ranges as stated earlier and seems to lack any physiological significance or to have any biological impact. Nevertheless, it would be interesting to do a similar study with subjects having glucose/ insulin problems (syndrome X, diabetes, etc.).

In relation to total cholesterol, there was a tendency toward reduction that did not reach

statistical significance. Although it should be pointed out that total cholesterol value for this sample population was within normal ranges. But when we separate the subjects with total cholesterol values of over 200 their mean total cholesterol value was 237.5 mg/dl $\pm$ 5.51 and at one week after treatment lowered to 211.05 mg/dl $\pm$ 5.25 which resulted in a statistically significant difference ($p<0.01$). In relation to triglycerides these reduced significantly after one week on the dietary treatment program. This dietary intervention program had no negative side effects, compliance was excellent (90%). A point of discussion is how can this short term program be effective. We believe is due to metabolic correction and systemic detoxification.

Metabolic correction refers to a combination nutrients that provides the necessary building blocks or cofactors to improve enzyme function. Thus, correcting and optimizing metabolism. These nutrients seem to correct subclinical deficiencies and metabolic imbalances probably due to a faulty diet consisting of empty calories

that lack the necessary nutrients and fiber. Also a faulty diet contains additives, processed material that may provide a toxic environment that may prevent or make difficult, the physiological changes necessary and metabolic alignment to achieve weight/ fat loss and at the same time assist normal physiological functions. The dietary supplement program presented herein resulted in a safe and effective short term way to achieve weight loss, reduce body fat and improve lipid profile.

References

(1) Gonzalez MJ, Miranda-Massari JR, Ricart CM. **Effect of a dietary supplement combination on weight management, adipose tissue, cholesterol and triglyceride in obese subjects.** *PR Health Sci J 2004,23:121-124.*

(2) Wellman NS, Friedberg B. **Causes and consequences of adult obesity: health, social, and economic impact in the United States.** *Asia Pac J Clin Nutr 2002,(58):5701-709.*

(3) Stern CJ, Colditz GA. **The epidemic of obesity.** *J Clin Endocrinol Metab 2004,89:2522-2525.*

(4) World Health Organization: **Obesity: Prevention and managing the global epidemic.** *Report of Who consultation on obesity. Geneva; World Health Organization 1997*

Other References

1. Antidepressant induce cellular insulin resistance by activation of IRS-1 kinases (Molecular and Cellular Neuroscience
2. http://www.hsph.harvard.edu/news/press-releases/archives/2002-releases/press11202002b.html

3. Free Fatty Acids Induce JNK-dependent Hepatocyte Lipoapoptosis

CHAPTER 8

ABOUT THE AUTHOR

Jim Harper is a genius, at least in his own mind! Ok, I am having some fun here. As I stated earlier in the book I refused to except a publishing contract because I did not wish to write a book that could not really give helpful information and make the book be 300 pages long for the publisher. So, I am writing the About the Author myself.

This has been a fun and relaxing book to write and frankly I needed a break from the drug withdrawal research I tend to spend too many hours a day with. I don't want the reader to feel like I have not spent the time I should researching and writing this book but for me it was completely relaxing and a sort of vacation from life for a while.

Several years ago I was helping a friend that produced a rodeo event for the National Police Rodeo Association and I had the opportunity to talk with one of the bull riders. I asked him, "Whatever made you want to ride bulls?" His answer, "I work on the Vice Squad, Hollywood Division, and riding bulls is what I do to unwind after work." Living in the Hollywood vicinity at that time of my life I completely understood how riding wild bulls could be relaxing.

Not that I compare myself to that police offer in any way with what he was doing but for me in my own little world I can relate.

My background was telecommunications system engineer and business for several decades. In 1999, when I was trying to decide what I was going to do when I grew up, by chance some information about psychoactive drugs presented itself to me one day on my porch. I began just having a look at a few studies on antidepressants and I uncovered some things that the medical community had missed. A very long story short, I developed a natural way for people to get off psychoactive medication and other addictive drugs with little to no withdrawal side effects. Over 40,000 people have now used this method to become drug free.

In 2005, I founded a company Advanced DNA Testing to gather additional information of how the human body metabolizes medications and nutrients. In 2005, I was authorized as an expert witness regarding the use of DNA testing in a case in Los Angeles, County.

One of my published books has been used as a college text for Psychopharmacology Doctoral students at a major U.S. university.

Over the past 14-years I have lectured at universities and medical conventions where physicians, psychiatrists and allied healthcare providers receive their continuing education credits.

Enough about me. This book is about you and for you. There is Hope. There is a Solution. Your health is important not only for you but to your family and friends. Losing weight incorrectly can cause more problems down the road that I would prefer you to not have.

Don't give up hope. Don't let anyone tell you, you can't do it. This is your life, your body, your body and you are the one that needs to make the decision or change will never happen. At least a positive change.

Losing weight can be one of the most difficult things you ever undertake. Take it one day at a time and if you backslide you can and should restart tomorrow.

Sometimes we are presented with a life event or a life opportunity that we look back at in some point in the future and know the decision to act or not act had an impact on who we are, how we feel about ourselves. We all have several times we should have acted or we should have stuck with something and seen it to a conclusion. Here you are again. It is decision time. See it through this time, finish it, look at yourself in the mirror each day and smile and say "I am doing this."

www.ingramcontent.com/pod-product-compliance
Lightning Source LLC
Chambersburg PA
CBHW060007300526
45794CB00003B/1118